FREDDY GBENGBASSA
Godelieve ODIA NDAMI
Jean Bosco G. D. KETORO

ECONOMIC STATUS AND QUALITY OF LIFE OF OLDER PEOPLE IN THE DRC

FREDDY GBENGBASSA
Godelieve ODIA NDAMI
Jean Bosco G. D. KETORO

ECONOMIC STATUS AND QUALITY OF LIFE OF OLDER PEOPLE IN THE DRC

Evaluation of data from the Boto Health Zone/South Ubangi Province

ScienciaScripts

Imprint
Any brand names and product names mentioned in this book are subject to trademark, brand or patent protection and are trademarks or registered trademarks of their respective holders. The use of brand names, product names, common names, trade names, product descriptions etc. even without a particular marking in this work is in no way to be construed to mean that such names may be regarded as unrestricted in respect of trademark and brand protection legislation and could thus be used by anyone.

Cover image: www.ingimage.com

This book is a translation from the original published under ISBN 978-3-330-87920-1.

Publisher:
Sciencia Scripts
is a trademark of
Dodo Books Indian Ocean Ltd. and OmniScriptum S.R.L publishing group

120 High Road, East Finchley, London, N2 9ED, United Kingdom
Str. Armeneasca 28/1, office 1, Chisinau MD-2012, Republic of Moldova, Europe
Printed at: see last page
ISBN: 978-620-3-74465-1

DEDICATION

To our dear and loving wife Godelieve ODIA NDAMI
To the GBENGBASA family.
GBENGBASSA NZEGE MBOMBA Freddy

The concept of the elderly is complex because it refers to age, but also vulnerability.

The aim of this study was to assess the quality of life of elderly people in the Boto Health Zone, in South Ubangi Province.

Methodology

The data come from the survey of ten Health Areas in the BOTO Health Zone in 2023. A weighted sample was applied to select the Health Areas. Using bi-variate statistical analyses, we examined the risk of living in old age, difficulties in moving around and eating, as well as the use of different income-generating activities, and the mode of adaptation according to age and type of environment.

Results

Older people face many financial difficulties in the health zone under study, and when faced with these challenges, they most often rely on loans from relatives and family assistance. As a result, financial assistance from relatives is also less common in the area because of the poverty that is rife in the country in general and at provincial level in particular.

KEYWORDS: Economic level; Quality of life; Elderly people.

Conclusions

Elderly people are experiencing more financial difficulties and, above all, in our country there is no structure for the day-to-day supervision and care of these people, many of whom die quickly as a result of mobility complications and the virtual absence of retirement pension costs.

Contribution

While the existing literature on ageing focuses mainly on health vulnerabilities, our study draws attention to economic difficulties. Our work also contributes to research on mutual aid from family and friends, highlighting the fact that financial assistance from family or friends seems to be less widely used by older people in the Democratic Republic of Congo.

SUMMARY

The notion of elderly people is complex because it refers to age but also to vulnerability. The objective of this study was to assess the quality of life of elderly people in the Boto Health Zone, in the South Ubangi Province.

Methodology

The data comes from the Survey in ten Health Areas of the BOTO Health Zone in 2020. A weighted sample was applied to select the Health Areas. Based on bivariate statistical analyses, we examined the risk of living in old age, difficulties in moving around, eating, as well as the use of different income-generating activities, the mode of adaptation according to the age and type of environment.

Results

Elderly people experience a lot of financial difficulties in the health zone under study. When faced with these challenges, the elderly most often rely on loans from relatives, family helpers. Consequently, financial assistance from relatives is also less frequent in the area because of the poverty that is rampant in the country in general and at the provincial level in particular.

IN MEMORIAM

To our late Father, Mathieu GBENGBASA KETORO PENZIBANGA, who has left us suddenly;

To our late Mother, Anne Marie NGOMA MOSUKUSA, who left us just a short time ago;

To our late Great Sisters VANA GBENGBASSA NONO and GBENGBASSA SESE Mathilde, who died suddenly;

May the peace of our Lord Jesus Christ be in your resting places until the great Day of Resurrection.

ACKNOWLEDGEMENTS

Mr DGA of ANAPEX, Professor Henry GERENDAWELE NGBASE Professor John EKINA BONGONGO, PhD Ms YANGBANDA MONGAKALE Sabrina; Mr MBUYI KANKONDE Arthur; Mr DASE TELO Calvin.

EPIGRAPHY

The seeds of healthy ageing are sown early." "Like museums, libraries are a refuge from ageing, illness, death." "As soon as you start spying on your body, ageing has begun." "The younger you are, the more active your ageing.

Marguerite Yourcenar

ALREADY PUBLISHED

- ✓ *Impact of LLIN use on the prevalence of malaria in Democratic Republic of Congo.*
- ✓ *World Bank Financing and Poverty Indicators in the Democratic Republic of Congo "Historical Critique from 1970- 2013".*
- ✓ *Explanatory factors for early adolescent fertility in Yakoma, North Ubangi Province.*

TABLE OF CONTENTS

INTRODUCTION

The world's population is ageing, with the proportion of adults and elderly people increasing and that of young people decreasing. This phenomenon is linked to the reduction in family size and longer life expectancy. It is inevitable, unless we return to the large families of yesteryear, which is inconceivable in the long term because it would lead t o unlimited demographic growth. Demographic ageing affects the whole planet, but it is more or less advanced depending on the country. In the countries of the South, it is often only in its early stages, but is set to become very significant over the coming decades. And it will happen more quickly than in the North. In China, for example, the proportion of people aged 65 or over is set to rise from 7% to 14% in just 25 years, and in Vietnam, in 17 years, whereas the same doubling took more than a hundred years in France .[1]

Ageing will have a profound impact on societies, and will require increasing attention from decision-makers in the 21st[e] century. In the developed world, but also in many parts of the developing world, the proportion of older people in the population is increasing rapidly. Ageing is a mark of the success of the human development process, since it is the result of lower mortality (combined with lower fertility) and increased longevity. Ageing also creates new opportunities, which go hand in hand with the active participation of older people in both the economy and society in general. In these countries, particularly in the developing world where the number of young people is still growing rapidly, the economic climate is favourable to economic development.

Population ageing also poses serious challenges, particularly with regard to the financial viability of pension schemes, the cost of healthcare systems and the full integration of older people as active partners in the development of society. World Economic and Social Survey 2007 analyses the opportunities and challenges of ageing populations and aims to facilitate discussions on the implementation of the Madrid International Plan of Action on Ageing1 adopted by consensus by the Second World Assembly on Ageing on 12 April 2002. The Madrid Plan provides a framework for integrating the issue of population ageing into the international debate on development and for putting in place national policies capable of meeting the challenge of working towards the emergence of societies open to all ages. The plan focuses on integrating ageing into the international development agenda, promoting health and well-being into old age, and creating supportive and enabling environments for older people.

ISSUES

As changing demographics continue to take their toll, governments will need to review their policies. At present, many countries do not take into account the valuable contributions that older people continue to make. Senior citizens are people whose age is aged 65 and over.1 Globally, the proportion of older people is growing at a faster rate than other population groups. This change in the structure and proportion of the population has implications at local and national levels that can be managed through timely policy responses. For developing countries, including OIC countries2 , population ageing presents challenges such as the sustainability of pension funds, pressure on the provision of health and social services for the elderly, and employment opportunities adapted to the elderly. The United States of America is allocating 8.3 billion US dollars to improve the quality of life of seniors living with disabilities .[3]

Ageing is not synonymous with a poorer quality of life in France; the quality score does not change with age, and the more negative the score, the more quality of life is affected by physical, social, psychological and economic problems.[1]

In Africa, the majority of elderly people rely on their families, live close to them or live with descendants who can offer material, financial and emotional support, so the care of older people will continue to depend on forms of family solidarity.[2]

In Côte d'Ivoire, people aged 65 and over are disabled as a result of physical problems, and their low economic level means that they have a problem with care, which requires considerable financial resources.[3]

In the Democratic Republic of Congo, the 2015-2016 SNIS report states that the living conditions of elderly people in the BOTO Health Zone remain worrying. Out of 1,047 cases of death recorded in the community, 207 are adult patients, including 160 cases of people aged 65 and over. In this category, 7 out of 10 cases die of malnutrition within 48 to 72 hours, despite proper treatment. In a bid to improve their quality of life, the Health Zone (ZS) is organising the affiliation of a number of patients to its network. compulsory for senior citizens to join the mutual health insurance scheme. On the other hand, for those hospitalised at the General Referral Hospital, there is a subsidy in terms of sugar, maize flour and soya. Despite these efforts, the number of deaths linked to malnutrition among the elderly remains alarmingly high. Human beings are in constant interaction with their environment, and in order to improve their quality of life, they are constantly seeking to improve their environment so that it can better meet their needs. Researchers have been investigating the interaction between human beings and their environment for around thirty years, but it is only recently that research has intensified in this area. Not only are we trying to find out more about the interaction between human beings and their environment, but we are also trying to determine what types of environment are needed to make life easier for people with specific needs. Take, for example, the progress that has been made in recent years to improve access to public places for people with physical disabilities. Older people contribute to society in many ways, whether within their families, in their local communities, or to society more generally. However, the extent of these human and social resources, and the opportunities open to each of us as we age, will depend very much on one key characteristic: our health.

If people enjoy good health during these extra years of life, there will be few limits to their ability to carry out the activities they enjoy. If these extra years are dominated by a decline in physical and intellectual capacity, the implications for older people and for society could be far more negative. Although it is often assumed that increased longevity is accompanied by a longer period of healthy life, the evidence that older people today are in better health than their parents is less encouraging.The elderly are a group with specific needs and, given the rapid growth in this population, questions are beginning to be asked about the type of environment best suited to them. The changes associated with ageing manifest themselves in many aspects of their lives, including their physical, socio-economic and social condition and their mental well-being[1] . People's needs change as they get older, as does their interaction with their environment. Sometimes, because of specific problems such as physical health problems, older people's environment is not sufficient to meet their needs, and they have to change their living environment. Specialised institutions with different types of services are built to meet the physical needs of these people. Approximately 5% of the elderly live in such institutions. institutions. So what happens to the physically independent elderly? Where do they live and how do they interact with their environment? They can, of course, remain in the same environment for the rest of their lives, or change their living environment altogether. They can choose to live in an environment where people of different ages live, or live in an environment reserved for older people.

CHAPTER 1
DEMOGRAPHIC DETERMINANTS OF AGEING

Population ageing is a phenomenon that occurs when the median age of a population increases as a result of falling fertility and rising life expectancy. The first section of this chapter deals with fertility and life expectancy, the main determinants of ageing. The second section is devoted to the different concepts associated with ageing, while the third presents the different problems faced by the elderly.

SECTION 1. FERTILITY AND LIFE EXPECTANCY

1.1. Fertility

The fertility rate indicates the number of live births per woman in a country. To maintain a natural balance in the population, a replacement fertility rate of 2.1 children per woman is considered adequate. Although fertility rates above replacement levels indicate population growth, very high fertility rates can lead to socio-economic difficulties for families.

On the other hand, fertility rates below the replacement rate indicate an ageing population and a simultaneous reduction in size. As with very high replacement rates, low replacement rates can also result in an ageing population. This has socio-economic consequences that need to be addressed through public policy and institutional adaptations.

1.2 Life expectancy of the elderly

Since the 1960s, demographic studies carried out in various countries have shown that life expectancy has increased in developed countries, and this phenomenon is also beginning to be observed in developing countries, particularly in urban areas. In the 21ème century, people around the world are tending to live longer. An increase in life expectancy is a testament to advances in science and medicine as well as better nutrition, hygiene, healthcare, education and economic well-being.

SECTION 2. DIFFERENT CONCEPTS RELATED TO AGEING

This section presents the various concepts related to ageing dealt with in this book and the underlying literature.

2.1. Quality of life

The WHO defines quality of life as: "An individual's perception of his or her place in life, in the context of the culture and value system in which he or she lives and in relation to his or her goals, expectations, norms and concerns. It is a broad conceptual field, encompassing in a complex way a person's physical health, psychological state and level of independence, his social relationships, his personal beliefs and his relationship with the specifics of his environment .[1]

2.2. Third age

People who leave the world of work with socio-economic and psychological consequences are at a point in their lives when the inexorable process of ageing accelerates, with all that this entails in terms of health problems and dependency.[2]

The "**third age**": this expression seems to have been coined initially to designate the stage that follows adulthood. The use of the ordinal adjective (third) refers to the order of generational succession. Thus, anyone who has gone beyond the first two phases (youth and adulthood) could be considered to be in the third age. Although this term was used for a long time, it has fallen out of favour due to the increase in longevity and the distinction made between different stages in the ageing process (the expression "4^{e} age" is sometimes used).[3]

Elderly person": the preferred choice is the expression "elderly person", which is more neutral because it refers only to age and no limit is really established (flexibility). It is the term recommended by international texts .[4]

The generally accepted definition is that the population concerned is that aged 60 and over. In the French-language literature on gerontology, we often find the word "Ainés", which conveys an impression of respect and can be proposed as an alternative. In the more technical sections, expressions such as

The term "60+" or "80+" is used primarily to designate age groups. However, age as the limit of a stage in life is entirely relative and varies greatly from one context to another, depending on culture, living conditions that are not conducive to healthy, active ageing, or existing legislation (e.g. pension legislation).

2.3. Ageing

This is the set of physiological and psychological processes that modify the structure and functions of the body from middle age onwards.[1]

It is a slow, progressive and irreversible process that results f r o m genetic and environmental factors and depends on individual or collective life events .[2]

Ageing is the general effect of time on a biological organism. This process reduces the functional reserves of most physiological systems, making them vulnerable to many diseases.

Ageing": a concept used by international institutions to designate the process leading progressively to old age and death. It explains the process by which the world's populations have ever-increasing proportions of people over the age of 60. This concept is important if we are to understand that the course of life is characteristic of all living beings, that it is irreversible and that each stage of life depends on the previous stages. It is the "lifespan" approach that is now being promoted in international policy frameworks.

In addition to these terms, we could also use the word "old" or "vieille", which may be acceptable in everyday conversation but is unsuitable as technical language, and risks having a pejorative connotation depending on the culture.

The processes involved in senescence are still largely poorly understood and require further research into the biology of ageing. The physiological process of ageing occurs simultaneously but not necessarily in parallel with chronological age.

While longevity appears to be 'heritable' to a certain extent (20 - 30%), research into the genes involved in the ageing process is still in its infancy, and we are gradually discovering the importance of a number of physico-chemical processes of metabolic significance, and which therefore depend on the environment in the broadest sense of the term: ecological, climatic, dietary, hygienic and socio-cultural. The rapid increase in average life expectancy since the beginning of the century highlights the important role played by extrinsic factors (living and working conditions, nutrition, improved housing, heating, clothing and hygiene, and medical advances).

2.3.1. Types of ageing

There are therefore three possible types of ageing[1]

✓ the "successful" process, with no pathology, a low risk of developing pathology and a high degree of autonomy;
✓ the "normal" process without pathology but with risks of developing pathology;
✓ the "pathological" process marked by numerous risk factors, pathologies and/or disabilities that set in at a very early stage.

To this can be added the concept of "**active ageing**", which for the WHO (2002)[2] , is defined as "the process of optimising opportunities for health, participation and safety with the aim of improving the quality of life of older people throughout life" and "**healthy ageing**", which for the European "Healthy Aging" programme, which aims to establish recommendations for health promotion and prevention for older people based on a review of the literature, is defined as "the process of optimising opportunities for health, participation and safety with the aim of improving the quality of life of older people throughout life".[3] which aims to draw up recommendations on health promotion and prevention for the elderly based on a review of the literature, is defined as follows "the process of optimising physical, mental and social health to enable older people to be socially active without discrimination and to enjoy independence and a good quality of life".The literature on the elderly increasingly refers to the concept of Healthy Ageing. Inspired by the population approach, this concept has evolved over the years to encompass all the determinants of health, including individual risk factors and factors linked to people's environment. One of the many definitions of ageing, that of the Public Health Agency of Canada, presents it more or less as an aspect of health promotion, prevention and protection that focuses on the factors influencing the ageing of the population.

This concept also involves maintaining a good quality of life and preventing disability[1] . For Health Canada, healthy ageing is "a lifelong process of optimising opportunities to improve and maintain physical, social and psychological health and well-being, independence and quality of life, and to promote smooth transitions between different stages of life" .[2]

According to the Centres for Disease Control and Prevention[1] , healthy ageing is a process that promotes the development and maintenance of optimal physical, social and cognitive well-being. In a safe environment, this process is made possible by adopting healthy lifestyle habits and making appropriate use of preventive services designed to minimise the impact of specific or chronic health problems. The Organisation for Economic Co-operation and

Development (OECD, 2000), with a view to maintaining the prosperity of ageing countries, centres its definition of active ageing on the narrower notion of productivity. It approaches active ageing as the ability of people as they age to lead productive lives in society and the economy. These people then have the opportunity to make choices in the way they live, learn, work, enjoy themselves and care for others.

In Bryant, Corbett and Kutner's Model of healthy ageing (2001), healthy ageing is the result of a series of links between different aspects and can be summed up by the expression "Going and doing"2 (Figure 1). These words, which could be translated as 'moving and doing', evoke well-being, fulfilment and self-fulfilment. The proposed model stresses the importance of factors whose presence can positively shape older people's perception of their own ageing, and the fact that, conversely, the absence of these factors leads to a negative perception. There are four interrelated factors. The first, having a goal and meaningful activities to carry out, refers to carrying out activities of daily living, but also to the importance of exercising social roles. Having the skills required to meet the challenges that arise is another factor (e.g. mobility, good cognitive functions, absence of sensory problems). The loss of certain functions affects the lifestyle of older people at different levels and can lead to a negative perception of their ageing. On the other hand, having access to the right resources and services can promote a positive view of ageing by helping to compensate for losses and maintain healthy lifestyles. Finally, having a positive attitude, i.e. the motivation to engage in activities, is a determining factor in self-fulfilment, the main foundation of this model for healthy ageing.Fulfilment, based on these four conditions, is modulated by factors such as support, the person's ability to adapt and the possibilities for compensation in the environment.

Figure 1: Going and doing model for healthy ageing

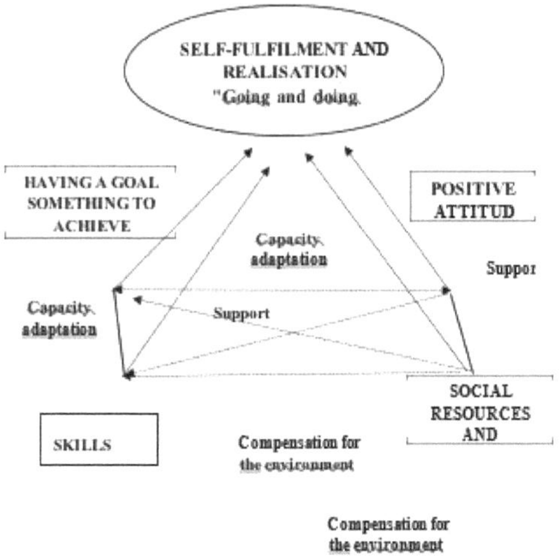

Taken from : L.L. Bryznt, Corbett and J.S. Kutner (2001). "In their own words: a model of healthy aging", Social sciences and medecin, 53 (7), p.927-941.

2.3.2. Vulnerable

A person is considered vulnerable when he or she is exposed to risks that are likely to push him or her into need or dependence on external intervention. Risk is defined as any uncertain event whose occurrence is unforeseeable and which may cause a shock likely to reduce, or even eliminate, the well-being of individuals, households or groups. Vulnerability refers to the risk of suffering the consequences of unforeseen events or shocks that could seriously affect well-being.

SECTION 3. PROBLEMS FACED BY THE ELDERLY

Seniors are often faced with health, physical, social, psychological and economic problems. In this section, we take a look at these different problems.

3.1. Health problems

The conditions most frequently reported by people aged 45 to 74 are dental problems, cited by almost nine out of ten people, and vision problems (refraction) (59%). Next come osteoarticular problems, cited by more than one in four. High blood pressure affects 11% of men and women. Sleep disorders and depression are also common. Seniors need both assistance with daily living and medical care. These needs fall broadly within the scope of social protection and social security: needs for social services and health services. What's more, they are not independent of each other. For example, care for the elderly is provided at the same time as medical care. It is therefore not always easy to differentiate between what is covered by health insurance and what is covered by a specific dependency system. The diversity of care systems therefore has a direct impact on care systems for the elderly, and the approaches taken by different countries in terms of The provision of care for the elderly is generally linked to the existing health (and more generally social protection) system.[1]

3.2. Physical problems

There are several: quality of pain, morbidity, current activities and leisure activities. In Belgium, the decline in the quality of life of the elderly is associated with a range of illnesses, risk factors (such as smoking, excessive alcohol consumption and obesity) and socio-demographic determinants; the problems most often reported concern the pain/discomfort dimension first, followed by mobility problems and problems in carrying out everyday activities. Finally, autonomy is the aspect least frequently reported .[2]

In Quebec, 87.5% of elderly people living in private households have no mobility problems; healthy elderly people who are economically advantaged and well integrated into their community spend more time at leisure and make less use of social and health services .[3]

In Switzerland, 45% of elderly people with a chronic illness feel that they do not have a good quality of life (compared with 25% for those with a chronic illness). among those who do not have a chronic illness). Fifty-eight percent of elderly people who are limited in their activities say that their quality of life is not good; 36% are limited but not very limited and 16% are not limited at all; more than three quarters of elderly people living at home - more men than women - say that they are satisfied with life in general .[1]

3.3. Social problems

Older people are faced with social isolation and relational difficulties. Advancing age has a number of social consequences, including a decline in social networks due to the frequent widowhood of women, the estrangement of children, the disappearance of contemporaries for the elderly, and a reduction in resources for many.[2] In France, 60% of elderly people are protected against the risk of dementia and cognitive decline by the presence of a social support network; 74% of elderly people no longer attend cultural and sporting associations .[3]

In Belgium, people in their third year of life benefit from standard home help services (meal delivery, personal hygiene care, assistance with home maintenance, etc.). Forty-four per cent of the elderly experience a negative feeling in the event of a sudden break in social relations; 45% of the elderly are well equipped socially and rely on a wide social network and do not feel alone .[1]

In England, 12% of older people say they have no children, reflecting their social and family isolation .[2]

3.4. Mental problems

People aged 65 and over present a number of psychological problems such as sleep disorders, self-esteem, negative feelings (despair, melancholy, anxiety, depression). And sex life. In France 50% of elderly people complain of insomnia, 30% hypersomnia and 15% sleep apnoea syndrome, 25% of Belgians aged 65 and over live with negative feelings such as melancholy, despair, anxiety and depression .[3]

In Morocco, 45% of older people have self-esteem that is positively associated with gender, place of residence, occupation, level of education and marital status .[1]

3.5. Economic problems

The economic problems of the elderly are the number of children in care, care in the event of illness, allocation of the large share of income, how to earn food, means of earning money, access to food and income-generating activities.

In Benin, older people work in the informal sector (men 10%, women 2%) and receive a retirement pension (men 52%, women 3%) .[2]

In Mali and Burkina Faso, 45% of elderly people living in poor households have difficulty accessing the food of their choice .[3]

In Cameroon, 50% of senior citizens derive their income from agriculture, livestock farming, trade and pensions .[4]
In the east of the DRC (Butembo), elderly people have difficulty accessing the food of their choice and the health services they need .[1]

3.5.1. Economic security for the elderly

Living conditions often deteriorate for the elderly. As people age, reduced economic opportunities and deteriorating health frequently increase their vulnerability to poverty. However, these conditions vary depending on the context and the category of older people. Means of subsistence tend to differ in the same way. In developed countries, pensions are the main means of existence and protection for the elderly, whereas in developing countries, few elderly people are entitled to a pension and must therefore find other sources of income. In fact, 80% of the world's population does not enjoy sufficient protection against health, disability and income risks in old age[2] . This could mean that, in developing countries alone, around 342 million older people do not currently enjoy sufficient income security. This figure could rise to 1.2 billion by 2050 if the coverage of current mechanisms designed to guarantee income security is reduced. the income of older people is not being broadened. The demographic transition poses an enormous challenge if we are to guarantee the existence and viability of pension schemes and other systems to ensure the economic security of an ever-increasing number of older people in both developed and developing countries. According to the conclusion of the survey on the situation in the world, this challenge is far from impossible to meet with appropriate measures.

3.5.2. Poverty among the elderly

Empirical evidence suggests that older people living in countries with universal pension and public transfer systems are less likely to fall into poverty than younger cohorts in the same population. In countries where pension schemes have limited coverage, poverty among older people tends to match the national average. Clearly, the likelihood of being poor in old age does not depend solely on pension coverage. As a general rule, the degree of poverty among older people varies according to level of education, gender and living conditions. The probability of falling into poverty among the elderly decreases as the level of education increases. Older women are more likely to be poor than older men. In developing countries, most older people experience enormous income insecurity when there is no formal pension scheme. For those who have no protection, often For small farmers, agricultural workers and workers in the informal sector, the notion of retirement does not exist. Having had no formal employment, these people are not entitled to a pension and, if they have not managed to accumulate sufficient reserves, they must continue to work in order to live. The situation can be quite precarious for the very elderly (aged 80 or over), who may not be as able to work as younger people. People in particular who experienced poverty at the peak of their working lives will remain poor, if they do not become even poorer with age.People who are above the poverty line but have not managed to save for consumption in old age are at risk of becoming poor as they grow older. Older people can often rely on family and community support to survive or supplement their income. In this respect, older people who are not married, who have lost their spouse or who are childless (especially women) are at even greater risk of severe poverty. Dependence on family networks may not fully protect older people from poverty, as these networks themselves have limited incomes. It is, of course, much more difficult to guarantee an adequate income for older people when poverty is widespread .[1]

3.5.3.Guaranteeing support for the elderly

To be able to lead a healthy, independent life in old age and participate in social life, older people need to be able to rely on care and support services, and these must be of high quality and affordable. Quality standards and the financing of care are regulated. This clarification is still pending. Care is a set of actions adapted to the needs, wishes and life situation of the person being cared for. Acts of encouragement are just as much a part of this as acts of kindness. Care takes into account both the resources and the limitations of the person being cared for. Care is a combination of supportive and caring actions. Depending on the life situation and fragility of the people concerned, action may focus more on stimulation, motivation, or even prevention and protection.[1] To ensure that acts of caring do not lead to dependency or guardianship, human dignity sets limits: caring actions must never undermine the integrity, self-determination, fundamental rights and respect of the person being cared for. It is important to bear in mind that autonomy and dependence are not contradictory Reinforcing positive self-concept. Person-centred action requires take into account the older person's self-concept. This is the person's self-image and how they evaluate it. This self-image is constantly changing. Because of their experience, however, older people have a well-established self-image. This stability can help compensate for missing skills. With age, it can also be an expression of reduced flexibility: the self-image we have learned to love can only adjust to a limited extent to age-related changes.

Care recognises the older person's self-concept and emphasises their resources, whether cognitive skills or practical day-to-day abilities. In this way, it avoids reinforcing negative aspects, such as the feeling of being incapable or useless. At the same time, care helps older people to adapt their self-image as much as possible to changes in their living conditions. Don't lose sight of the living environment.

A person-centred approach means always taking account of the environment in which the person lives. New challenges and changes in the spatial, social and institutional environment are the starting point for developing mastery skills and strategies. Above all, it's about understanding the other person's experience, way of thinking and feelings. Person-centred work means finding solutions and means together with the people concerned, and not at the expense of others. their place. Taking charge does not mean executing, but making[1] possible.

CHAPTER 2
POPULATION AGEING IN THE DRC

The demographic ageing of a population occurs when the population structure shows proportionally few young people and many elderly people.

SECTION 1. AGEING IN RDC

In the Democratic Republic of Congo, an analysis of demographic statistics from 1984 to 2000 shows that the population of the Democratic Republic of Congo (DRC) is not very old, is not ageing and is dying rather young. It turns out that the DRC is not following the demographic pattern that characterises the industrialised countries of Europe, which are experiencing a population trend known as the demographic transition, starting from a given situation of low population growth due to a high birth rate and high mortality, and ending up in a situation still characterised by low population growth, but this time caused by low mortality and birth rates. In the DRC, despite a relative fall in mortality, fertility is not declining, but is even increasing. The result is an age structure that is getting younger and younger and less and less old. The author proposes two kinds of action: action to enable the population to age (to combat premature mortality) and action to reduce the number of old people. not getting too young (promoting responsible parenthood), and those aimed at ensuring support for the elderly.[1] According to data from the Demographic and Health Survey (EDS-RDC, 2013-2014), the proportion of older people (aged 60 and over) is 4% of the population as a whole, and there is virtually no difference between the sexes (4% for men and women), or between places of residence (4% in urban and rural areas)[2] . This supports the hypothesis that "the Congolese population is not very old, it does not age and it dies rather young".

Figure 2. Age pyramid of the Congolese/Zairian population in 1984.

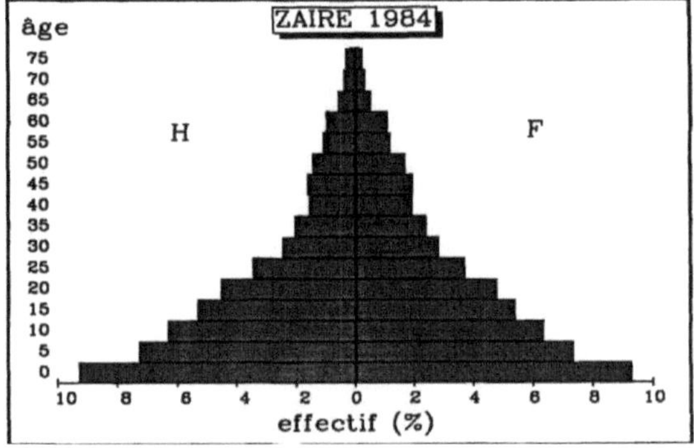

Source: INSS-RDC, General Population Census, 1984

The figure below clearly shows that there are fewer people aged 65 and over, around 4%. The pyramid with a widening base and a narrowing top.

Figure 3. Age pyramid of the Congolese population in 2014.

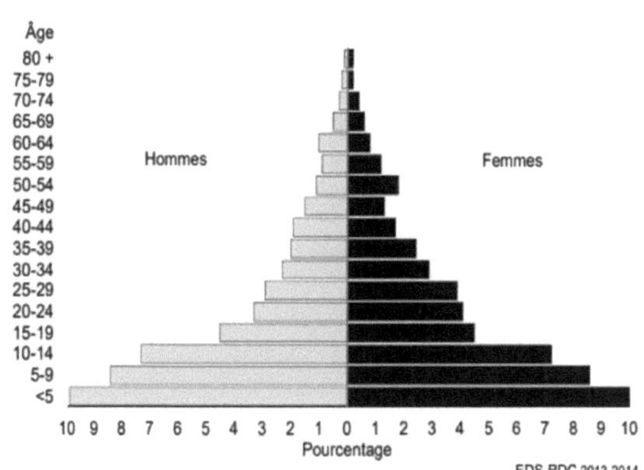

Source: Demographic and Health Survey (EDS 2013-2014).

Several years later, the situation remains unchanged. When we compare the two age pyramids, we see that even though here we are starting with people aged 65 and 80 plus, the proportion remains the same at 4%. The pyramid has a wider base and a narrower top.

SECTION 2. MANAGEMENT OF AGEING IN RDC

The social dynamics and mechanisms used to care for elderly dependents in the Democratic Republic of Congo are very different from those in developed countries. Very few elderly people have access to a pension, and they are disconnected from the few health facilities that provide care. (one is a public institute; the other looks after pensioners from the civil service and certain private sectors). In the Democratic Republic of Congo, no law has been passed to provide free care for people over 60, as is the case in Senegal and other countries. In particular, certain services in health facilities are free of charge.Families are increasingly stepping in to make up for the State's shortcomings. However, these families, who are also economically and socially vulnerable, have to be inventive to mobilise the resources needed to care for their elderly and sick relatives.

Sometimes, assistance is segmented and fragmented according to the capabilities of each family member. Often, in addition to financial care, the day-to-day management and support is also divided. The women look after their husbands' washing and the older daughters look after their mothers'. The men of the family take care of accompanying their parents to health facilities or, failing that, paying for treatment.

It should be noted that some elderly people continue to meet their own expenses and even those of their children. In health institutions, these carers are called upon to feed their parents if they are in hospital, or to help them with exercises during physiotherapy sessions. This work continues at home with massage sessions and rehabilitation exercises. These carers In the end, these families develop the knowledge and skills that we refer to as lay knowledge. Mastery of these 'skills' gives them a privileged status, in the same way as those who pay for medical care or family expenses, and enables them to avoid paying for care. The role and place of family carers in the care of dependent elderly people in the Democratic Republic of Congo highlights the power relationships between individuals within the family, as well as the positioning games played by these actors in their quest for social status.

2.1. Health and social protection systems

Dependent people need both assistance with daily living and medical care. These needs fall broadly within the scope of social protection and social security: needs for social services and health services. What's more, they are not independent of each other. For example, dependency care is provided at the same time as medical care. As a result, it is not always easy to distinguish between what is covered by health insurance and what is covered by a specific long-term care system. The diversity of care systems therefore has a direct impact on dependency care systems, and the approach taken by different countries to dependency care is generally linked to the existing health (and more generally social protection) system.

2.1.1. Health and social protection systems in the DRC

In the Democratic Republic of Congo (DRC), the vast majority of the population has no form of social security. Few people have a regular job or receive a salary. The majority work in the informal sector, earning irregular and unstable incomes. It is therefore the ability to pay that determines access to healthcare, in particular by relying on family solidarity. Social security cover in the formal sector is poor, and only applies to civil servants and employees of a few companies.

Because of a low tax base (due to the importance of the informal sector), weak institutional capacity for tax collection (inadequate administrative coverage of the territory), and non-compliance with tax laws, financing a healthcare system through tax collection (the

Beveridge system in Great Britain) is therefore difficult. We could take inspiration from the Bismarckian system, based on contributions from workers and employers.

In order to achieve this, the population needs to be made more aware of the concept of health insurance, so as to instil in them a spirit of foresight: "contribute for the day when you fall ill". This will avoid emergency expenditure, which is often the cause of delays in access to care. Although the State cannot finance this social security system in its entirety, as legislator it must nevertheless be able to organise and regulate the sector and improve the general conditions of access to healthcare. Universal health insurance, such as exists in Europe, seems out of reach for the time being in the DRC. Mutual insurance (a voluntary, not-for-profit insurance structure) would seem to be a good system for a proportion of the population capable of paying regular contributions, in particular salaried employees and civil servants. Private mutuals (profit-making organisations generally reserved for the wealthy minority) cannot represent a solution for the majority of the population. The State must remain in charge, in particular by: (1) providing an appropriate environment for the promotion of mutual societies within the meaning of the Mutuality Act (2) regulating the private insurance sector, including by passing laws requiring them to cover low-income people and defining the minimum cover that such insurance must offer beneficiaries (e.g. cover for emergencies) (3) promoting access to health services for lower-income groups through subsidies and the elderly .1

2.1.2. Social protection in the DRC

Social Protection refers to all the collective welfare mechanisms that enable individuals to cope with the financial consequences of social risks, i.e. situations likely to compromise the economic security of individuals or their families, by causing a reduction in their resources or an increase in their expenditure. On the one hand, it enables individuals to survive when they are hit by social risks, secondly, to reduce inequality in the face of life's risks, while ensuring a minimum income to enable them to integrate into society.[1] The extension of Social Protection is one of the priorities of the International Labour Organisation (ILO)[2] and is the main focus of the Government of the Democratic Republic of Congo, which is working to extend effective Social Protection cover to all sections of the Congolese population by 2030. The starting point for this is to guarantee a minimum level of Social Protection to the majority of the population through the establishment of a Social Protection base in the form of social mutuals.

2.1.3. Mutual insurance social

These are "groups which, mainly through their members' contributions, aim to carry out, in the interests of their members and their dependants, a welfare, mutual aid and solidarity scheme to prevent personal social risks and compensate for their consequences".[3]

Social mutuals operate on the basis of the following principles:

✓ voluntary and non-discriminatory membership;

✓ not for profit ;

✓ democratic and participatory operation ;

- ✓ commitment to solidarity ;
- ✓ autonomy and independence ;
- ✓ volunteering ;
- ✓ responsibility.

Health mutuals, which are widespread in the DRC, are a form of social mutual insurance that covers the financial risks associated with illness.

CHAPTER 3

ECONOMIC SITUATION OF THIRD AGE PEOPLE IN THE BOTO HEALTH ZONE

In this chapter, we will describe the socio-demographic characteristics of the elderly in the health zone, describe the characteristics of the household where the elderly live, describe the economic and financial situation, and determine the quality of life and dependency of the elderly in the health zone under study.

SECTION 1. SOCIO-DEMOGRAPHIC CHARACTERISTICS

In this section, we will present the elderly according to sex, age, marital status, religion, level of education and occupation.

1.1. Breakdown of senior citizens by gender and socio-demographic characteristics

The data relating to this proportion is presented in the table below.

Table 1. Proportion by gender according to age, marital status and religion of the elderly.

AGE	SEX	MALE	FEMALE			TOTAL
	n	%	n	%	n	%
65-69	87	47	98	53	185	41,7
70-74	66	55	54	45	120	27
75-79	22	34,4	42	65,6	64	14,4
80-84	22	53,7	19	46,3	41	9,2
85-89	9	47,4	10	52,6	19	4,3
90-94	5	45,5	6	54,5	11	2,5
95 and over	3	75	1	25	4	0,9
Single	10	Mat status 83,3	rimonial 2	16,7	12	2,7
Married	147	79,5	38	20,5	185	41,7
Widower	41	18,6	179	81,4	220	49,5
Divorced/separated	16	59,3 Religion	11	40,7	27	6,1
Catholic	131	47,3	146	52,7	277	62,4
Protestant	78	49,4	80	50,6	158	35,6
Kimbanguist	1	33,3	2	66,7	3	0,7
Revival Church	3	100	0	0	3	0,7
Jehovah's Witnesses	1	50	1	50	2	0,5
Neo-apostolic	0	0	1	100	1	0,2
Total	214	48,2	230	51,8	444	100

Table 2. Proportion by gender according to school attendance, level education and occupation.

Attendance school Male Female	Gender of senior citizen				Total	
	n	%	N	%	n	%
Yes	128	81	30	19	158	35,6
No	86	30,1 State level	200 ude	69,9	286	64,4
No level	3	2	00	00	3	1,9
Primary	93	59	27	17,1	120	75,9
Secondary	21	13	3	1,9	24	15,2
Normal	11	7 Profession	00	00	11	7
No	80	37	136	63	216	48,6
Sale of salt and alcohol	2	28,6	5	71,4	7	1,6
State agent	11	100	00	00	11	2,5
Agriculture	55	45,5	66	54,5	121	27,3
Hunting	16	88,9	2	11,1	18	4,1
Trade	8	53,3	7	46,7	15	3,4
Breeding	16	59,3	11	40,7	27	6,1
Chikwangue	00	00	2	100	2	0,5
Mat and Graba making	15	100	00	00	15	3,4
Sentinel	11	91,7	1	8,3	12	2,7
Total	214	48,2	230	51,8	444	100

1.2. Proportion of third-year students by school attendance

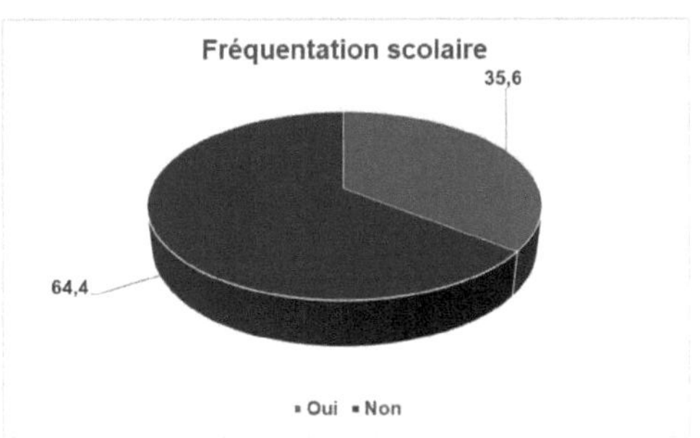

Figure 4: School attendance among the elderly.

1.3.Breakdown of elderly people according to Household characteristics.

The data from table below show these characteristics.

Table 3. Presentation of data on household characteristics.

Occupancy status of the plot Sex of the elderly person

Total MaleFemale						
	n	%	N	%	n	%
Owner	146	73,4	53	26,6	199	44,8
Tenant	2	50	2	50	4	0,9
Underhoused	37	20,1	147	79,9	184	41,4
Lodged by the employer	18	60	12	40	30	6,8
Family home	10	43,5	13	56,6	23	0,9
Home for the elderly	1 Size of	25 house hold	3	75	4	100
1,-5	77	51	74	49	151	34
6,-10	80	45,5	96	54,5	176	39,6
11 and more 57 Status in household or live		48,7 60 people from		51,3 third	117 age	26,4
Head of household 162		74,7	55	25,3	217	50
Relative of head of household32		18	146	82	178	40,1
Brother-in-law or mother-in-law of the head of8		30,8	18	69,2	26	5,9
Friend and acquaintance of the1		50	1	50	2	0,5
Son of head of household0		0	2	100	2	0,5
Other to be specified 8		57,1	6	42,9	14	3,2
Total 214		48,2	230	51,8	444	100

1.4. Breakdown of elderly people by quality of accommodation by gender

The table below shows data on the quality of housing by sex for the elderly.

Table 4. Quality of housing by sex of senior citizens

Sex of the elderly person Housing quality Total Male Female						
	n	%	N	%	n	%
Very dissatisfied	11	57,9	8	42,1	19	4,3
Dissatisfied	48	48,5	51	51,5	99	22,3
Neither satisfied nor unsatisfied	22	59,5	15	40,5	37	8,3
Satisfied	127	45,2	154	54,8	281	63,3
Very satisfied	6	75	2	25	8	1,8
Healthy environment						
Not at all	62	50	62	50	124	28
A little	102	47,7	112	52,3	214	48,2
Moderately	35	49,3	36	50,7	71	16
Many	14	41,2	20	58,8	34	7,7
Extremely	1	100	0	0	1	0,2
Total	214	48,2	230	51,8	444	100

1.5.Breakdown of senior citizens by condition economic and financial data by gender

The table below showsthe data on this breakdown.

Table 5. Proportion of senior citizens by economic and financial conditions

Number of children in burden	Sex of elderly person Male	Female			Total	
	n	%	N	%	n	%
1,-5	77	51	74	49	151	34
6,-10	80	45,5	96	54,5	176	39,6
11 and over	57 Activi ty	48,7 income-generating	60	51,3	117	26,4
Trade	7	50	7	50	14	3,2
Breeding	22	62,9	13	37,1	35	7,9
Agriculture	61	45,9	72	54,1	133	30
Family transfers		37,5	5	62,5	8	1,8
Chase	9	81,8	2	18,2	11	2,5
Sentinel	12	92,3	1	7,7	13	2,9
Pension/retirement costs	2	100	0	0	2	0,5
No	74	37,2	125	62,8	199	44,8
Others to be specified	24 Support	82,8	5 de maladi	17,2 e	29	6,5
Myself	92	73	34	27	126	28,3
My husband or wife	16	53,3	14	46,7	30	6,8
My children	86	34	167	66	253	57
My grandsons	6	40	9	60	15	3,4
Others to be specified	14 Satisfaction with state of health	70	6	30 nity	20	4,5
Very dissatisfied	24	53,3	21	46,7	45	10,1
Dissatisfied	132	47,3	147	52,7	279	62,8
Neither satisfied nor dissatisfied	16	38,1	26	61,9	42	9,5
Satisfied	42	53,8	36	46,2	78	17,6
Total	214	48,2	230	51,8	444	100

1.6. Breakdown of elderly people by current quality of life, by sex

Data on the quality of senior citizens is presented in the table below.

Table 6. Proportion of senior citizens by current situation, by gender.

Les 4 situations suivants laquelle correspondent mieux à votre situation actuelle	Sexe de la personne de troisième âge				Total	
	Masculin		Féminin			
	n	%	n	%	n	%
Vous mangez tous les aliments souhaitez	4	50	4	50	8	1,8
vous mangez tous à votre faim mais pas toujours les aliments que vous souhaitez	151	47,8	165	52,2	316	71,2
il vous arrive parfois de ne pas avoir suffisamment à manger	49	46,7	56	53,3	105	23,6
il vous arrive de rien trouver à manger	10	66,7	5	33,3	15	3,4
Etes-vous satisfait(e) de vos relations avec les autres						
Très insatisfait(e)	3	25	9	75	12	2,7
insatisfait(e)	39	43,8	50	56,2	89	20
Ni satisfait ni insatisfait	20	50	20	50	40	9
Satisfait	152	50,3	150	49,7	302	68
Avez-vous souvent l'occasion de pratiquer des loisirs						
Pas du tout	116	44,1	147	55,9	263	59,2
Un peu	58	50	58	50	116	26,1
Modérément	31	62	19	38	50	11,3
Beaucoup	9	60	6	40	15	3,4
Sécurité dans votre vie quotidienne						
Pas du tout	39	54,9	32	45,1	71	16
Un peu	87	50,9	84	49,1	171	38,5
Modérément	42	45,2	51	54,8	93	20,9
Beaucoup	46	42,2	63	57,8	109	24,5
Total	**214**	**48,2**	**230**	**51,8**	**444**	**100**

1.7. Distribution of elderly people by means of transport and ability to carry out the tasks of daily living, by gender.

This breakdown is shown in the table below.

Table 7. Proportion of elderly people by mode of transport and ability to perform tasks of daily living, by gender.

How do you manage Sex of the elderly person Total Move Male Female						
	n	%	n	%	n	%
Very difficult	63	44,7	78	55,3	141	31,8
Difficult	106	48,4	113	51,6	219	49,3
Fairly easy	33	51,6	31	48,4	64	14,4
Easy	12	60	8	40	20	4,5
Satisfaction with ability to perform tasks of daily living						
Very dissatisfied	54	43,2	71	56,8	125	28,2
Dissatisfied	112	45,9	132	54,1	244	55
Neither satisfied nor dissatisfied	15	51,7	14	48,3	29	6,5
Satisfied	33	71,7	13	28,3	46	10,4
Total	214	48,2	230	51,8	444	100

SECTION 2. INTERPRETATION OF RESULTS

The main objective of this study was to assess the socio-economic level and quality of life of elderly people in the Boto health zone in the province of Sud Ubangi in the Democratic Republic of Congo.
The data from our study show that the average age of these patients was 72±7 years, with a predominance of the age group aged 65-69, or 42%. More than half of senior citizens lived alone (widowed/divorced/separated, single), i.e. 58.3%.
What's more, two-thirds of the subjects in this study (64%) had not attended school, and of those who had, three-quarters (76%) were at primary level. Older people whose childhood dates back to colonial times have benefited little from schooling, due to the lack of school

infrastructure that is as varied and better distributed across the provinces as it is today. To this should be added the lack of interest shown by the population, which at the time was unaware of the benefits of education imported from the West. Most parents preferred to have their children accompany them to the fields or hunting grounds rather than let them go to school. This situation could go a long way towards justifying the high illiteracy rates and low education rates observed among the elderly in the Boto health zone. With regard to plot occupancy status, it is important to note that almost half of the elderly were owners of the plot they occupied (45%). Less than half were heads of household or relatives of heads of household (40%), and two-thirds cohabited with between 6 and 11 people in the household. In the majority of cases, polygamy was common among men, who forced elderly people to marry young women and own plots of land. On the other hand, the elderly women were all housed by their children. In terms of the number of dependent children, two-thirds of the subjects (66%) had 6 or more dependent children. In the Health Zone, orphans or children of single mothers are generally entrusted to their grandparents, who are obliged to take on the role of parents again despite their advanced age. In addition, the men had children from marriages with young women. They were forced to work hard to ensure the survival of their families. From a social point of view, older women in Africa want to live with their families. A study by Esther Cristelle Eyenga Dimi, 2011, in Cameroon showed that 50.5% of women aged 65 and over had more than 5 children to support, with children who were orphans or the offspring of single mothers being entrusted to their grandparents, forcing them to take on the role of parents again, despite their advanced age.As for the quality of their accommodation, two-thirds of the third-age people were satisfied with their homes (63.3%) and just over three-quarters were not completely satisfied with their surroundings (76.2%). The dwellings of the people under study were in the care of their sons, sons-in-law or grandsons and were regularly maintained, but these sometimes eccentric dwellings were surrounded by weeds.

In addition, 28.3% of care in the event of illness is provided by the elderly themselves. This meant that the elderly had to work hard, as part of their income was allocated to their own needs and those of their descendants, while other parts went towards schooling, clothing and health insurance for their children and grandsons. In terms of food, over two-thirds (71.2%) of the elderly ate their fill, but not always the food they wanted. Food was either prepared at home after their young wives returned from the field, or came from other family members. As for sources of finance, more than half of the subjects in this study had at least one income-generating activity, 55%, and the multiple burdens borne by them and the virtual absence of a retirement pension <1%, obliged the elderly in the area to create income-generating activities despite their advanced age. In most Central African countries, a good number of elderly people often set up income-generating activities (agriculture, fishing and trade), points out Annes Loones in her work carried out in Cameroon in 2008.

On the other hand, the proportion of elderly people who had difficulty with mobility was 81%, and the proportion who were unable to carry out the tasks of daily living was 83.2%, which proves the dependence of elderly people on other members of the community for food, housing, mobility or the ability to carry out the tasks of life and care in the event of illness.Other literature, such as that by Joceline Camiran et al, 2012 in Quebec, has shown that elderly people have an inability to be mobile or to carry out the tasks of everyday life; similarly, Rana Charafendinne, 2014, in Belgium, in her work, has added dependence on other people to those mentioned above, for Dr Jean Pierre Aquino, 2013 in France showed that older working people were unable to carry out the activities of life, although these three studies were carried out in developed countries.

BIBLIOGRAPHY

A.B. et al, "Etat de santé et environnement siciodémographique d'un groupe de groupe de personnes marocaines âgées", Colloq. Int. Meknès Maroc, 17 to 19 March 2011, n°2005,p. 100- 105, 2011.

A.C.T. épse SAY. "Les conditions de vie des personnes âgées en Côte d'Ivoire : Regard sur la maltraitance à Adjame Village", Colloq. Int. Meknès Vkieil, la Population. Dans les pays du Sud, n°2006-2007, p.29-35, 2011.

PUBLIC HEALTH AGENCY OF CANADA, site visité en January 2006.

AMADOU SANNI. M., "Les défis urbains du vieillissement au Bénin", Proceedings of the Meknès International Colloquium, p.13, 2011.

AQUINO.J-P., Anticipation pour une autonomie oréservée : un enjeu de société, " J.Artic., p.132, 2013.

ARTICLES 3 and 4 of Presidential Decree 05/176 of 24 November 2005 creating the National Social Protection Support Programme.

BACRO. F., and FLORIN.A., " Entre complexité et richesse : la diversité des défis liés à l'intérêt des chercheurs et des professionnels pour la qualité de vie " ; La Qualité de vie, Fabien Bacro, n°32eme APSLF, pp.7-12, 2014.

BRYANT, L.L., K.K. CORBETT and J.S. KUTNER (2001). "In their Social science and medicine, 53(7) 927-941.

C.D. MATHERS and others, "Global patterns of healthy life expectancy in the year 2002", BMC Public Health, vol. 4, no 66.

CARLO KNÖPFEL, Guide to good care in later life Clarification of terminology and guidelines, 2014, p5.

CARSAT Bourgogne-Comité, "Cahier des charges du thématique sommeil version 2017", IMPA, p.1-16, 2017.

Centers for Disease Control and Prevention - Research Centers Healthy Aging Network, 2006.

COMMITTEE ON AGING AND SOCIETY. (1988). The social and built environment in an older society, Washington D.C., National Academic Press.

D.S.S. KOUASSI. Conditions de vie des personnes du troisième âge dans une Afrique en récession économique : Le cas du Cameroun, Article, pp.3-4, 2007.

D.ZIMMERMANN-SOUTSKIS, F. MOUREAU-GRUET, and E. ZIMMERMANN, Comparaison de la qualité de vie des personnes âgées vivant à domicile ou en institution OBSAN Report 54. 2012.

ECE DIMI, "Situation socio-économique des personnes âgées au Cameroun Etat des lieux et facteurs explicatifs Esther, "Colloquium. Int. Meknès Maroc, 17 to 19 March 2011, n° 2005, p.412-430, 2011.

GEORGES MUSAVULI, in Butembo (DRC), Prise en charge des personnes du troisième âge, p.1 -10, 2011.

GILLES PISON, Le vieillissement démographique sera plus rapide au Sud que au Nord, Bulletin mensuel, d'information de l'institut national d'étude Démographique, 2009

HEALTHY AGING - DRAFT report (2006).

I.L.P.N.N.S(PNNS), 2011-2015, "Nutrition and dietetics - foods for special dietary uses", J. Artic, pp.303-405, 2014.

ILO Recommendation 202 of 2012

LAURENCE ASSOUS and PIERRE RALLE, La prise en charge de la dépendance des personnes âgées : une mise en perspective internationale, Helsinki, 25-27 September 2000.

LOONES.A., and E.D.-A.P. JAUNEAU, "La fragilité des personnes âgées : Perceptions et mesures", J. CREDOC, p.36-37, 2008.

M-A. DELISTE, "Les loisirs des personnes âgées : tendances actuelles et perspectives d'avenir", J.Artic, p.15-342, 2005.

MINISTRY DES AFFAIRS DE ACTION

HUMANITARIAN AND SOLIDARITY, strategic plan action plan for the elderly 2017-2021.

MUNDABI. MA. What social security system for the DRC: HEALTH INSURANCE? Mutuelles? Assurances privées, Conseil -Assurance Maladie, Paris (France).

UNITED NATIONS, World Economic and Social Survey 2007, sustainable development in a world of globalization. ageing overview, Business Department economic and social.

NGONDO a PITSHANDENGE, SERAPHIN, Du vieillissement de la population en RDC: état de la question, mécanismes explicatifs, facteurs de promotion et propositions de stratégies, 1990.

OIC, Organisation of Islamic Cooperation

WHO (World Health Organization), Active ageing: Geneva: WHO, 2002.

P. BREUIL-GENIER "Aides aux personnes âgées dépendantes: la famille intervient plus que les professionnels" Economie et statistique, n° 316-317, (1998a).

PASCAL.L., "Evaluation de la qualité de vie des personnes âgées diabétique en Seine-Maritime, 'U.F.R DE MEDECINE- PHARLACIE DE ROUEN' (France), 2014.

Madrid International Plan of Action on Ageing National Social Protection Policy, Vol. 1, December 2016.

DRC, Ministry of Planning, Demographic and Health Survey (EDS 2013-2014), INSS, 2014.

United Nations resolutions 45/5 of 16 October 1992 and 48/98 of December 1993; see also communication material for the International Year of Older Persons 1999.

ROBINS et al, Autonomie des personnes âgées, ARS Poitou-Charenets, vol.155,11, 2014.

ROSSO-DEBORD.M.V., "par la commission des affaires en conclusion des travaux de la mission sur la prise en charge des personnes âgées dépendant", 2010.

ROWE JW. and KAHN RL. Successful aging. The Gerontologist, 1997, 37: 433-440.

RUTTEN.P, "Soutenir les liens sociaux de la personne âgée dépendante pour une vie de qualité à domicile", Rennes, France, 2003.

S.V. et Al, Vieillir, mais pas tout seul, Fondation. Belgium

Health Canada, 2001. Workshop on Healthy Aging. Part 1: Aging and Health Practices. Ottawa: Health Canada.

SCHOUMAKER. B., "Ageing in sub-Saharan Africa", Espace. Popul. Soc, vol.18, n°3, pp.387-388, 2016.

SYLVAIN. H. " Analyse de la qualité de vie des personnes âgées dépendantes, inscrites au réseau gérontologique de la Haute saintonge", 2014.

T.L.L and GERY.Y., "Promouvoir la santé des personnes âgées", Hist. Médecine société, vol.401, 2009.

CONTACT

Freddy Gbengbassa Nzege Mbomba *is a doctoral student in the evaluation of development programmes and projects. He is head of research at the University of Kinshasa (UNIKIN) and the Institut Supérieure Pédagogique de la Gombe (ISP/GOMBE). He is currently Assistant to the Director General of the Agence Nationale des Promotions des Exportations* ***(ANAPEX)****.*

He is also a UNESCO Statistician/Statistician for Action Research on Measuring the Learning of Beneficiaries of Literacy Programmes - ***RAMAA II-RDC****, at the UNESCO Institute for Lifelong Learning* ***(UIL)/Germany****.* ***Address****: Rue. KINDUTI, n°05/Binza Ozone/ Ngaliema/Kinshasa/République Démocratique du Congo.*

E.mail : freddynet3@gmail.com

*Telephone****: +243 84 25 96 395/ 81 651 58 43***

Ageing populations create support needs that are less and less met by public services. It is therefore relevant to explore the coping strategies used by older people to meet the challenges they face, by comparing them with other age groups.

The concept of the elderly is complex because it refers to age, but also vulnerability.

The aim of this study was to assess the economic level and quality of life of the elderly in the Boto Health Zone, in the South Ubangi Province.

What's more, their quality of life remains precarious due to the lack of economic support for the elderly from the Congolese state.

In the DRC, it is difficult to know the situation of the elderly, as there has never been a general census of the elderly. Most of them are abandoned to their own devices.

***Freddy GBENGBASSA NZEGE MBOMBA** is a PhD candidate in the Evaluation of Development Programmes and Projects. An expert demographer by training, he is currently Assistant to the Director General of the Agence Nationale des Promotions des Exportations **(ANAPEX)**.*

*He is also a statistician at UNESCO, responsible for **RAMAED-RDC** statistics.*

*He is responsible for teaching the Data Collection and Analysis and Project Evaluation, Ethics and Professional Conduct courses. professional.... at the Institut Supérieur Pédagogique de la Gombe **(ISP/GOMBE)**.*

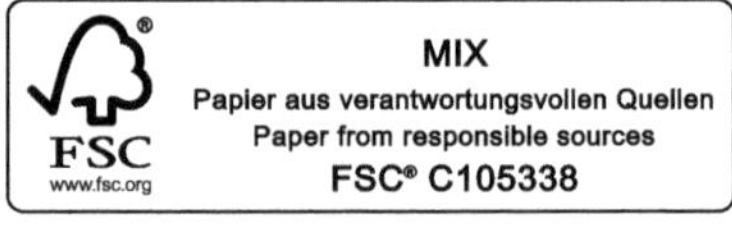

Printed by Books on Demand GmbH, Norderstedt / Germany